DIET REVOLUTION

The Ultimate Guide
to Help You Get Healthier New You
with Balanced Meals

Weight Loss Guaranteed

by

Betty Smith

Thank you for purchasing this book. No part of this book may be reproduced, scanned or distributed in any manner without written permission from the author, except in case of brief quotations used in books, articles or newspapers. Your support and respect for the property of this author is appreciated.

This publication contains the opinions and ideas of its author. It is sold with an understanding that the author is not engaged in rendering medical, health or any kind of personal professional services in this book.

The ideas and suggestions in this book are not intended as a substitute for consulting with a physician. This book is intended as reference only, not as a medical manual. The author shall not be liable or responsible for any loss or damage allegedly arising from any information or suggestion in this book. Mention of specific companies, organizations or authorities does not imply endorsement by the author, nor does mention of specific companies, organizations or authorities imply that they endorse this book or the author.

Copyright © 2017 Betty Smith

All rights reserved.

ISBN-13: 978-1718812536
ISBN-10: 1718812531

CONTENTS

INTRODUCTION

It's not a short-term diet. It's a life style change.

This book is for those who are looking for an eating plan that will help them lose weight (guaranteed) and is sustainable for life.

I'm not a doctor. I'm just like you - if you picked up this book, you are in a place I used to be — a busy woman with family and responsibilities, overwhelmed by daily stress and information, and often contradictory on how to get back on track and regain healthy weight.

Growing up, I was blessed with a slim and healthy body. I was very active and would have never thought I'd have weight problems in the future. Right after college, when I got my dream job with its demands and long hours, slouching over a desk, my body started to change. I started packing on pounds. Within a year I didn't recognize myself. One day, after not being able to look at myself in the mirror, I decided to take back control of my weight; and that is how my weight loss journey began.

Within the next year I had tried pretty much all the programs and diet plans available, only to fall back into my old habits shortly after. After a lot of trial and error, I finally came up with an eating plan that produced results and was relatively easy to stick to. I'm very happy to share my experience in the hope that it will help numerous people, struggling daily, feeling alone and discouraged. Forget about counting calories, starving yourself and daily weighing! However, this plan does require some discipline. After all, you can't achieve any significant results without doing actual work.

I would like to stress that all of the diets available have close to zero long-term success rate. The reason for this is simple: permanent weight loss requires a life-style change. But don't be discouraged – it's not an impossible task! You just have to keep at it daily until it becomes a habit. I've been there, I've done it and so can you (and I'm definitely not a poster man for a strong willed person).

In this book I will talk about diet a lot. But not the "diet" you normally think about. Nowadays, this word has a very negative connotation, when in fact it really means "the way we eat". To be healthy, you have to stick to a healthy diet. Not a fad diet that will slow down your metabolism and bring back your pounds with their "friends" right after you stop. Healthy doesn't mean starving – ever. Healthy means eating the right foods and being active. You have to follow a diet rich in all essential nutrients, minerals and vitamins that are necessary for us to function with optimal health and weight.

In this book I've shared the basic principles I've learned throughout the years that will help you get back on track and reach your weight loss goals. If you follow them, you won't be starving, feeling deprived or listless. Although you will most likely feel hungry in the beginning (generally our hunger is physiological and our body craves foods we are so used to eating), it will get easier with time and soon you won't even miss the old "diet". Remember, it takes 21 days of healthy eating and being active for it to become a habit. Now, let's get started!

STOP COUNTING CALORIES AND EAT MORE

We all know that a sure way to lose weight is to consume fewer calories than we spend: eat less and exercise more or eat less than our daily needs and see stubborn pounds disappear. We need to count calories to know how much food we really consume. Health experts recommend it, celebrities do it, and our friends who lost weight do it… However, counting calories does not save you from eating disorders and their consequences; furthermore, counting calories can turn into a disorder in itself. To find a true balance and to succeed on your journey you need to stop calculating the calorie count of every bite that you put in your mouth and start eating healthy foods as that is the only way to achieve your dream health goals. This chapter is all about the need to eat a balanced diet to automatically adjust the calorie count. So read on!

What Happens When You Count Every Calorie?

When you start obsessing over packages of food for the calorie count, you stop paying attention to what is actually within the package. You start adding up the calories, making up the daily-recommended calorie count and ignore the fact that you need healthy food on your plate, not numbers. Let's suppose your daily-recommended calorie count is 1,500. You might end up fulfilling that need from proteins and carbs only and neglect to add healthy fats. Thus, weighing every single crumb of food can potentially do more harm than good (and it often does).

Why Is Counting Calories a Bad Idea In the First Place?

The first and foremost reason for putting down your calculator and notebook is that the labels on the food packages are commonly misleading and can make you consume more or fewer calories than the figures displayed on the labels. Another reason is that counting calories is not an exact indicator of weight gain or weight loss. The calorie count of the foods varies by the season; for example, sweet tomatoes in the summer contain more calories than the pale ones in winter. Furthermore, not all calories that we consume are absorbed by the body, thus the actual calorie intake differs from the one that actually becomes a part of our body. Another important reason is that when you start counting calories, your diet becomes extremely limited. If your calorie needs are fulfilled by consuming meat, bread, milk and eggs, you would see no reason to add fruits, nuts, raw veggies, and fish to your diet. The essential nutrients, present in these foods, fail to become a part of your daily diet and a deficit of these vital nutrients may arise, making you prone to a myriad of health disorders. Your obsession with numbers will bring no benefit whatsoever.

What You Should Do Instead.

Give up the math and concentrate more on eating real food. Start eating more healthy fats, proteins, and carbs in proportionate amounts. Stop meddling with the body's natural balance and give it proper fuel to work so that weight-regulating mechanisms kick in. When your diet becomes balanced, your body automatically starts losing extra pounds, eliminating the need to count calories for losing weight. Here is what you can do to make your diet better.

- **Listen to your body (really)**

This should be your new mantra. Instead of stopping when your calorie count is up, stop when your tummy is almost full, so that your starved body gets its share of much-needed energy. Be extremely aware of mindless eating. I like to approach eating almost as a meditation: no distractions (TV, cell phones, etc.). Eating with family members and friends is an added bonus – when you engage in great conversation you eat slower and thus, you get full faster. Always keep portion size in check and don't serve food in family style portions. A great trick that always works for me is using a colored medium-size plate (the darker the color the better). Dark colors make the plate look fuller so you trick your brain into thinking you have eaten more. Big white plates require lots of food to fill them up and it's very easy to overeat. So it's not always a lack of will power or discipline that makes you eat more but simple things like the color and the size of your plate! Another helpful tip to keep in mind: never eat snacks directly out of the bag. We have all heard about portion control and we've seen those little pre-packaged snack bags. However, you know you get more savings when grocery shopping for a family and trying to stay within budget by buying food and snacks in big packages. Just be sure to put your chips or popcorn into a small serving dish and the rest – out of sight. Otherwise, you won't even notice how you got through that huge bottomless bag of chips, popcorn or candy!

Eat properly spaced meals and avoid skipping breakfast or lunch, so you don't become famished by the end of the day and stuff yourself.

- **Flavor up your diet**

Stop denying yourself the sweet pleasures. Don't indulge in sugars, though! Go for complex carbohydrates that don't break down instantly but take longer to digest. Those are the ones to opt for. Complex carbs are found in pasta (yes, you can enjoy pasta in moderation; in fact, some pasta sauces are more harmful than pasta itself, because they contains too much refined sugar), whole grains, soy products (organic and in moderation), dairy products, etc.

- **Eat more fats**

You heard that right! Consuming healthy fats is imperative to maintaining healthy weight. Especially important is consumption of omega-3 fats, which are found in rich quantities in fish like salmon, trout, etc. Avoid trans-fats, like those found in baked goods, margarine, fried foods, etc. According to the latest studies, we shouldn't fear saturated fats found in coconut oil and butter. These fats are good for you! Also, eat more unsaturated fats, like the ones present in essential oils (olive oil) and nuts. Unsaturated fats are good for your heart as they prevent clogged blood vessels, thereby averting development of cardiovascular disorders.

You also need to build up your fat stores, so that during a hunger state your body relies on fat for energy consumption instead of proteins. This way, fat stores are cut down and muscles become chiseled, making the bulk of your muscles stand out.

- **Eat good proteins**

These are the ones that have low fat content. Don't limit yourself to eggs and meat only to fulfill your calorie needs. Nuts, yogurt, cottage cheese, seafood, lentils, peanut butter, and beans are all rich sources of lean proteins. Proteins are crucial for building up muscle mass and for carrying out vital cellular processes.

- ## Go green

Fresh, raw vegetables and fruits are rich sources of a wide variety of nutrients, minerals, and vitamins that contribute towards regulating your metabolism and help in achieving ideal body mass index. It's best to aim for organic if you can afford it or have access to local farmer's market, but don't stress over it too much. Any produce is better than no produce!

- ## Mix, blend, and vary

Don't stick to the same recipes and ingredients. Alter your dietary patterns as much as you can, keeping above recommendations in mind. I included some of my favorite super easy recipes in this book, however, don't stop there either. Look for and try different variations to treat your taste buds every now and then. It is the only way to provide your body with much-needed carbs, proteins, fats, vitamins, and minerals in balanced amounts, while enjoying your food.

So What Happens When You Count Less And Eat More?

As the nutrient levels of your body reach their optimal concentration, your metabolism starts working at its full potential, burning off calories as they are consumed, storing the needed amount and shedding off the rest of them. The metabolism runs faster when provided with fuel to run it. The result is an optimal health state in which body stores only the essential amounts of fat, as well as a lean body frame with less fat and more muscles. Your overall health will improve dramatically once your body reaches that perfect balance between calorie consumption and calorie burn-off due to a boost in metabolism.

The only thing that you need to do is relax around food and everything will fall into the right place by itself. Pay attention to the food, not the numbers; that is the ultimate tip for healthy eating and healthy living.

SUGAR TRAP: THE HIDDEN CAUSE OF WEIGHT GAIN

Less fat, more exercise and you'll be all set to lose weight overnight, they say. What they forget to add to the list is sugar – often the real culprit behind weight gain. Sugar silently wreaks havoc on your system and if you are trying to lose weight or maintain good health, it is the sugar you need to watch out for more than the fat.

What kind of sugars must be avoided, what kind should be consumed? This chapter is all about the silent sugar traps you might unknowingly fall victim to. I have been a sugar addict myself for many years. I gained the most weight when I fully gave in to my sweet cravings. At one point I was eating 4-5 Great American cookies a day, not knowing they each have 350-500 calories. Just these cookies alone comprised more than my daily calorie allowance and I thought I was just snacking or eating dessert! Not to mention, they are loaded with sugar and bad fats! If you have a sweet tooth and consider indulging in sweets to be an innocent snack – pay attention.

The Ugly Truth About Sugars

Sugars are either simple or complex. Simple sugars are not that simple, though. Since they are already in simple (refined) form, they don't need to be broken down any further and are readily absorbed into the blood stream and utilized for production of energy. The excess amount of simple sugars is converted into glycogen and stored in the adipose (the fat tissue located in the liver and muscles), hence contributing to an increase in the fat stores of the body.

Complex sugars, on the other hand, need to be broken down into simple sugars before they can enter the blood and be transported to cells. This prolonged digestion time makes them ideal for long-term energy provision. Also, since sugars are slowly broken down and absorbed, the body utilizes what sugar is available to it in simple form. Slowly, complex sugars break down and are absorbed, and by the time they are completely digested, little is left for conversion into glycogen.

Another fact to keep in mind about refined sugars is that they do not alleviate hunger. They only increase food cravings because they have little effect on satiety centers in the brain as compared to complex carbohydrates. Less stimulation of satiety centers will leave you hungry even after consumption of large amounts of foods that contain refined sugars.

Sugar is also highly addictive. A lot of new research suggests that it is as addictive as cocaine and I'm sure a lot of us will agree! This is due to the fact that consumption of simple sugars causes release of large amounts of dopamine in the neuronal circuits, especially the "reward center" of the brain, leaving us feeling better than before. As a result, people who have a tendency to become addicted can become hooked onto sweet foods. The food industry knows this and they are doing everything they can to keep us hooked: sugar is added to yogurt, chips, pasta sauces, ketchup, and salad dressing – foods it should never be in! It's used in a whopping 75% of packaged foods purchased in the US. The latest statistics show that the average American consumes anywhere from a quarter to a half pound of sugar *a day*! We're talking mainly about added sugar here. Natural sugar sources like whole fruits and vegetables are not very concentrated as the sweetness is buffered by water, fiber, and other nutrients. Also, how many fruits and vegetables does the average American consume? Not as many as they need to. So comparing sugar to drugs makes a lot of sense. To produce sugar, natural whole foods like beets are stripped of their water, fiber, vitamins, and minerals to produce purified sweet stuff. All that's left are pure, white, sugary crystals. Similar refinement processes transform other plants like poppies and coca into heroin and cocaine. Refined sugars also affect people's bodies and brains. Those of us who love sugar are all too familiar with its drug like properties: cravings, withdrawal, and feeling of a reward ("sugar high"). Sugar stimulates brain pathways just as an opioid would and has been found to be habit-forming.

Consumption of sugar in large amount and high body fat content can lead to insulin resistance. Insulin is the hormone that is responsible for lowering sugar concentration in the blood. Insulin resistance contributes towards many diseases, including obesity. Therefore, it comes as no surprise that sugar causes rapid weight gain, especially in adolescents. Sugar is more dangerous than fats when it comes to weight gain. So avoid it as much as possible and go for complex sugars instead.

Fat Free = More Sugar = Weight Gain

Many times, you reach for the "fat free" labels at the supermarket not knowing that you are succumbing to a ruse. People have, after all, more fat-phobia than anything else. What you don't know is that removal of fat from food products takes away their taste. So to add taste to these foods, more refined sugars are added. More refined sugars serve only to make you fatter. Beware of these "zero percent fat content" labels, for they are nothing but marketing schemes, meant to trick you into buying those food items and are completely unhealthy.

The truth is that sugar hides in the most unlikely foods that are generally perceived as being healthy, but are secretly waiting to fatten you up. This is why eating healthy foods and maintaining normal body mass index at the same time has become such a challenge. It is better to know about these hidden sugar traps to be able to avoid them.

<u>Here are some of the foods that are likely to fool you:</u>

- **Salad dressing**

The creams added to the salad dressings are nothing but sugar in disguise. While you are busy eating fruit or vegetable salad and congratulating yourself for eating healthy, the sugar is busy piling up fat in your body.

- **Fruit juice**

Fruit juices are another kind of horror story. The general notion about fruits is that they are healthy, and they are – in a raw form. Fruits contain large amounts of fructose, which is another simple sugar and is otherwise known as "fruit sugar". Fructose is, however, harmful only in large amounts; fructose overload does not happen with eating only fruits. Fiber and water content of fruits make them resistant to easy digestion.

When pulp and fiber are taken out of these fruits, the fruit juice left behind contains nothing but fructose. The additives generally added to fruit juices also contain large amounts of sucrose and fructose. Fructose is broken down by the liver, and when the liver is already loaded with glycogen, it converts fructose into fat thus increasing body's fat content. It is, therefore, better to avoid fruit juices and just eat more fruits.

- **Processed food**

Processed food is just as healthy as junk food. During processing, this food is deprived of its nutrient content, leaving behind nothing but fat, refined sugar, and preservatives. Take strawberries, for example. Half a cup of strawberries contains 3.5 grams of sugar while strawberry ice cream has 15 grams. You can eat almost five times as many strawberries without compromising your health.

- **Breakfast cereal**

Who would suspect something as innocent as cereals to contain sugar? But yes, they do contain sugar as additive, so watch out!

- **Meat sauces and chicken spreads**

It might look like you are stocking up on protein. What you don't know is that you are also consuming sugar that is added to these sauces and spreads.

- **Fruit yogurts**

Not only do they contain processed fruits, they are also full of sugar additives that are meant to sweeten them up. Don't fool yourself that you're eating a healthy yogurt; you're only pouring sugar into your body.

- **Peanut and almond butter**

You need to think twice before eating that peanut butter for it is not just protein that you'll be eating but also large amounts of sugar. Choose sugar-free varieties only!

- **Pasta sauce**

Everyone knows that spicy sauce accompanying spaghetti contains proteins and veggies. Did you know that it contains a sizeable fraction of sugar too? Most of these red sauces contain large amounts of refined sugar.

- **Chocolate milk**

It's not just plain milk. It's a mixture of humungous amounts of sugary additives and sweetened chocolate. Don't overload yourself with sugar just for a moment of sweet pleasure.

The Bottom Line

These hidden sugars cause more damage than fat in equal amounts, so be vigilant and look after your diet, otherwise you will fall a victim to this sugar trap. Avoid these food substances and go for their healthier alternatives before it's too late. Replace sugars with honey, for instance. Use homemade sauces and spreads instead of the sugar-loaded packaged sauces that you buy. Our diet and health are in our own hands; let's take good care of them while we can.

WHY THIS PROGRAM WORKS:

Your New Friend Fat,

The Power of Protein

And The Right Carbs

In The Right Amount

Of all approaches I have tried, the basics of Atkins diet made the most sense to me. This is why its principles are at the basis of my life-long program. If I have told you that you can shed all those extra pounds by reducing the intake of bread, pastries, and sweets while still indulging in bacon, nut butters, and tofu, it would sound weird, right? That is, however, the truth. Low carbs combined with high fat and protein intake, otherwise known as the "Atkins diet", is one of the fastest ways of losing weight. The idea behind this dietary regime is not to cut down the carbohydrate intake altogether and consume as much fats and proteins as possible. Rather, it focuses on the consumption of the right kind of nutrients in the right amount.

Following are the numerous health benefits that come in the wake of the diet Atkins pattern and the advantages of individual dietary components in the right amount.

What Is the Atkins Diet?

Bent on solving the problem of his increased body weight with diet only, late Dr. Robert Atkins introduced a dietary regime in the 1960s that was to alter people's lives for years to come. The diet was based on the simple principle of consuming the right kind of dietary nutrients in the right amount. This diet aims at cutting down the intake of carbohydrates to a minimum while at the same time increasing the intake of fats and proteins. Carbohydrates are severely restricted during the initial stages only and are progressively eaten in higher amounts until the desired weight goals are reached. This plan is easy to maintain since starting at the last stage and going forward you are eating a lot of carbohydrates (good ones, of course), so you don't feel deprived.

The idea behind the Atkins diet is pretty simple. The body utilizes carbohydrates as its primary source of energy but when the intake of carbs is restricted, the body turns towards alternative energy sources – the fat stores of the body. The accumulated fats are metabolized, generating ketones during the process that are utilized for fueling the body. As the fat stores come under attack, the body weight returns to normal. Low levels of carbs and high levels of proteins cause early satiety and reduce appetite. As a result, you will automatically eat less. This is why this dietary pattern is ideal for rapid weight loss. Atkins diet also helps regulate blood glucose levels, improve insulin sensitivity, and help prevent obesity.

The diet has been designed to help you stop counting calories and focus more on the actual diet. Over recent years, many researchers have established the efficacy of low carb, high fat and protein diet in reducing weight. The Atkins diet has been widely acclaimed as one of the most successful weight loss strategies. It has been deemed more effective than a low-fat diet. It is healthier than a low-fat diet, as our bodies do need more fat than we were taught to believe. As we know now, good fats along with omega-3s are essential to our physical and mental well-being.

The entire dietary regime is divided into four phases:

- **Phase I (induction)**: less than 20 grams of carbs per day mostly from low-carb veggies. This dietary pattern is known as "ketogenic diet".
- **Phase II (balancing)**: nuts, low-carb vegetables and small amounts of fruits are slowly added to the diet.
- **Phase III (adjustment)**: still more carbs are added until weight loss slows down.
- **Phase IV (maintenance)**: intake of maximal amount of healthy carbs for maintenance of body weight.

There is no hard and fast rule to follow these phases in order, though. Most people overlook the induction phase. They choose to go straight to the second phase instead and this is fine if you are a carb lover like I am. The length of each phase depends on your desired weight loss. I would recommend between 2 weeks and 1 month for Phases I and II (Phase II will usually be longer, especially if you need to lose more weight) and transitioning to Phase III after you're within 10 pounds of your desired weight (you can transition sooner if you're ok with a slower progression).

Friendly Fats

To understand what kind of fats you are allowed to consume, it is first important to understand the concept of good and bad fats. Good fats are unprocessed fats that are naturally found in foods. These include avocados, flaxseed, coconut and olive oils, eggs, and nuts (almonds, peanuts, walnuts, etc.). Especially important among these natural fats are the omega-3 fats that are typically found in fish like sardine, salmon, trout, etc. Oils and fats may be saturated or unsaturated. For decades, unsaturated fats were believed to be superior to saturated fats, owing to their beneficial effect on heart and blood vessels, but recent studies have shown saturated fats to be equally good. When someone brings up the topic of saturated fat your mind probably immediately goes to the thought of avoiding it because it "causes obesity". We have basically been fed the lines about how we need to avoid saturated fat because it causes heart disease, obesity, and other complications. While an excess of saturated fat may be linked to those types of illnesses, it's not the only culprit nor does it play as much of a role as we once thought.

Before we get into the nitty gritty of it all, you should first know exactly what saturated fat is. When you think of saturated fat, burgers, French fries, potato chips, and the likes come to mind. Talking from a chemical standpoint, these fats are composed with no double bonds between carbon molecules. Instead, they are saturated with hydrogen molecules to even out the bonds; hence where the term "saturated" fat comes from. Because of this molecular structure, the fats are usually solid at room temperature.

Because we've been lectured on the importance of avoiding this fat for years, it used to be a huge no-no in our diet. Many studies have shown the link saturated fat has to heart attacks, heart disease, obesity, and some other diseases. However, many of these studies have since been proven wrong with new, more accurate research. If you remember highly controversial Time's cover story "Eat Butter", published in 2014, it stated that scientists were wrong about saturated fats after all. There's no evidence to support the notion that saturated fat causes heart disease. Now, if that is confusing you – don't get discouraged. Below, I'll present compelling arguments for you to make your own conclusion.

Many populations eat a diet high in saturated fats and aren't plagued with diseases we are battling now, so the evidence in favor of saturated fats is becoming overwhelming. Bad fats are the ones that have been processed by hydrogenation, more widely known as "trans fats". They are more commonly present in packaged food items like chips, cookies, fast food, etc. They are bad for the reason that they tend to block the arteries, thus reducing the blood flow to the heart and brain therefore increasing the risk of heart problems and stroke. Refined vegetable oils like soybean, safflower and corn oil contain trans-fats and should be avoided at all costs.

When it comes to obesity, those who have put on the extra pounds were thought to be consuming too much saturated fat. One of the most recent studies by Hooper L, et al. "Reduction in saturated fat intake for cardiovascular disease", Cochrane Database Systematic Review, 2015, found no statistically significant effects of reducing saturated fat, regarding heart attacks, strokes or all-cause deaths[1]. This was a systematic review and meta-analysis of randomized controlled trials, performed by the Cochrane collaboration, an independent organization of scientists. The test included 15 randomized controlled trials with over 59,000 participants. Each of these studies had a control group: reduced saturated fat, or replaced it with other types of fat. It lasted for at least 24 months and looked at hard endpoints, such as heart attacks or death. Although reducing saturated fat had no effects, replacing some of it with polyunsaturated fat led to a 27% lower risk of cardiovascular events (but not death, heart attacks, or strokes). The surprising conclusion was that people who reduced their saturated fat intake were just as likely to die, or have heart attacks or strokes, compared to those who ate more saturated fat. That's right. Saturated fat did not increase the risk of obesity or heart disease at all.

Another study by Schwab U, et al. "Effect of the amount and type of dietary fat on risk factors for cardiovascular diseases, and risk of developing type-2 diabetes, cardiovascular diseases, and cancer: a systematic review", Food and Nutrition Research, 2014, found that consuming saturated fat was not linked to an increased risk of heart disease or an increased risk of type-2 diabetes[2]. It included 607 studies, randomized controlled trials, prospective cohort studies and nested case-control studies. Participants included both, people who were healthy and those with risk factors. The researchers found that partially replacing saturated fat with polyunsaturated or monounsaturated fat may lower LDL cholesterol concentrations and decrease the risk of cardiovascular disease, especially in men. However, substituting refined carbs for saturated fat may increase the risk of cardiovascular disease.

And a third important study Chowdhury R, et al. "Association of dietary, circulating, and supplement fatty acids with coronary risk: a systematic review and meta-analysis", Annals of Internal Medicine Journal, 2014, reviewed cohort studies and randomized controlled trials of the link between fatty acids and the risk of heart disease or sudden cardiac death[3]. The study included 49 observational studies with more than 550,000 participants, as well as 27 randomized controlled trials with more than 100,000 participants. The study did not find any link between saturated fat consumption and the risk of heart disease or death. So, people with higher saturated fat intake were not at an increased risk of heart disease or sudden death. Furthermore, the researchers did not find any benefit to consuming polyunsaturated fats instead of saturated fats. Long-chain omega-3 fatty acids were an exception, as they had protective effects.

After all we've been told about how saturated fats are bad for us and with new research bringing about the actual benefits of saturated fats, are they really the enemy that they have been made out to be for so long? In fact, in another study, it was discovered that women who consumed more of this fat in their diet actually lost more weight. This is due to saturated fat inhibiting the production of lipoprotein – which correlates with a risk of heart disease and weight-gain. This is why when saturated fat was first introduced to the world as being harmful and the cause of weight gain, obesity rates actually went up as people avoided it in their diets.

Good fats cause an increase in the levels of high-density lipoprotein (HDL) cholesterol within the body while reducing the amount of low-density lipoprotein (LDL) cholesterol at the same time, which is advantageous to a cardiac profile. Also, the cholesterol myth is suffering greatly lately. In 2012, researchers at the Norwegian University of Science and Technology examined the health and lifestyle habits of more than 52,000 adults ages 20 to 74, concluding that women with "high cholesterol" (greater than 270 mg/dl) had 28 percent lower mortality risk than women with "low cholesterol" (less than 183 mg/dl)[4]. Researchers also found that, if you're a woman, your risk for heart disease, cardiac arrest, and stroke are higher with lower cholesterol levels.

We should also keep in mind that certain fats and their ratios are more crucial than others. Omega-6 and omega-3 are essential fatty acids that you have to get through your food. Many western nations have too big a ratio between omega-6/omega-3, which can be the actual cause for many diseases and illnesses that are overly present in those communities.

While the optimal ratio of omega-6/omega-3 is still under consideration due to needed levels differing from person to person, a lower ratio is unanimously more beneficial. The truth is that most people in western societies have too much omega-6 in their system while they aren't getting enough omega-3s. A ratio that is high in omega-6 has even been linked to heart disease. The bottom line is that there isn't a correct ratio for omega-6/omega-3 yet. However, there has been ample evidence that shows that lower ratios have been the most beneficial when it comes to your health.

So, good fats are your new friends now! As you might have guessed, my favorite types of fat that I love to indulge in are Greek yogurt (plain), avocados, real butter, artisanal cheese (in moderation), and coconut oil added to soups, tea (and coffee if you drink it) or over steamed vegetables and side dishes.

By now, you must be thinking, how much fat do I need? Almost 30% of your calorie intake should be derived from fats. This should include saturated, monounsaturated and polyunsaturated fats in balanced proportions. Extra virgin olive oil is a rich source of monounsaturated fat. You should consume roughly 16 grams of saturated fat (for a 2,000-calorie diet) daily to be considered healthy. The best sources of saturated fat are foods like meat, whole-fat dairy foods, coconut oil, eggs, chocolate, fish oils, some nuts, and butter. Go for plant-based fats more than animal fats for they are more beneficial. High amounts of fat are necessary to reduce food cravings as a fat-based diet is more filling and appeases the hunger by slowing down the release of glucose in the blood. Also, it enhances burning of stored fats. In summary, you need to eat fat to lose fat, isn't it great?

The Power of Protein

Proteins are the basic building blocks of the body. They are needed for building various body structures, for enzymatic reactions, hormonal functions, neurotransmitter synthesis, and much more. Proteins also play a significant role in accelerating weight loss. In contrast to fats, though, they act on glucagon (produced in the pancreas). Among the effects of glucagon is its ability to release fat stores. Proteins are also more filling, compared to carbohydrates as they reduce appetite. According to a recent study, consumption of low carb/high protein foods in one meal is likely to lessen the food intake during the next meal by 5 percent.

Nutritionists recommend protein intake to be ½ grams per pound of body weight, which is far too little considering the fact that the protein requirements vary from one person to another. An athlete needs higher proportions of proteins as compared to an inactive person. Protein requirements of pregnant women are also higher. The Atkins diet calls for consumption of at least 6 ounces of (weighed uncooked) protein in a single meal: this is the starting reference point I have chosen for myself.

Whey protein, soy protein, sodium and calcium caseinate are important proteins that must be incorporated into the diet, according to the Atkins diet. Proteins are obtained from foods including poultry, fish (salmon, trout etc.), lamb, beef, eggs, butter, soy products, essential oils, etc. High fat protein sources like sausages, bacon, and hot dogs should also be avoided, focusing more on lean meats. Protein bars and shakes are also a good way of ensuring high quality protein intake. Several studies indicate plant-based proteins to be more effective compared to animal proteins.

An important question about proteins comes up for vegetarians. According to a number of recent studies, we can fulfill our protein needs by consuming plant-based foods only, so I'd recommend listening to your body and its needs. Don't starve yourself and definitely don't skip your yearly doctor checkups to ensure optimal health!

Curb the Carbs

The recommended daily allowance for carbohydrates for people following the Atkins diet is 20 grams per day in the beginning, with progressive increase in the amount of carbs being consumed. This carbohydrate requirement is fulfilled from non-starchy vegetables, butter, cheese, cream, etc. Pasta, grains (wheat, rice, barley, etc.), bread, high carb vegetables (carrots, turnips, etc.) and high carb fruits (bananas, apples, oranges, etc.) intake is not recommended. Sugary foods like ice cream, sweets, cakes, fruit juices, soft drinks, etc. should be avoided altogether.

How low is low carbs, after all? The simple answer to this question is: as low as it can be. A strict control over carb intake has to be exercised. The lesser the carb intake, the better the health and weight-loss benefits would be. Due to the restricted intake of fruits, vitamin and mineral levels within your body are also bound to drop, for which vitamin and mineral supplements are recommended. Don't get discouraged – such a strict carb regime is temporary to ensure your successful weight loss! You will be able to slowly reintroduce your favorite carbs.

Following this dietary regime means strict control over your cravings, so while keeping a close eye over your weight, you have to control sweet temptations. Not all sweets are banned, though. You are still allowed to indulge in chocolate, cream, and cheese, etc.

The Benefits of Low Carb, High Fat, and High Protein Diet

The benefits of the Atkins diet extend far beyond weight loss only. Let's have an overview of the major pros and cons that you are likely to face when embarking on this journey.

Pros

• The major benefit that the Atkins diet brings to its followers is that it is pretty easy to follow, given the fact that not all the culinary pleasures are denied. You can still enjoy your favorite foods like chocolate, cheese, cream, etc. This is in sharp comparison with other dietary regimes, making it an easy-to-follow diet.

• Speedy weight loss is one of the biggest advantages, especially for people who are overtly conscious of their body weight and image. It is due to the fact that fat stores come under direct attack, molding the body into a slim figure. There have been anecdotal reports of as much as 80% decrease in the body weight following strict adherence to the Atkins diet.

- There is no danger of becoming underweight. As the Atkins diet plan is divided into stages in which the amount of carbohydrate intake is slowly increased until the ideal body weight is reached, and the person learns what the ideal amount of carbohydrates is that they need to consume in order to maintain their body weight. This is what makes the Atkins diet stand out from other dietary regimes that severely restrict the calorie intake to have people end up as skeletons, instead of reaching their dream weight goals.

- The Atkins diet has been especially proven to be beneficial for people suffering from epilepsy as it decreases the risk of seizures in such patients. Its efficacy has been proven through rigorously held clinical trials in epileptic patients. These patients have been reported to have complete seizure-free intervals when kept on a low-carbohydrate/high fat and protein diet for some time.

- Since the fat stores of the body are depleted, the risk of fat deposits as plaques in the blood vessels (atherosclerosis) is reduced. Atherosclerosis is the main culprit behind the clogging of blood vessels and subsequently reduction of the blood supply to the vital organs like brain and heart. In this way, the risk of major cardiovascular diseases like stroke, angina, coronary heart disease and heart failure is reduced. This is one of the greatest health benefits of the Atkins diet.

- A low carbohydrate diet regulates the levels of insulin in the body, thereby enhancing the insulin sensitivity. The incidence of diabetes, especially type-2 diabetes, is therefore significantly reduced.

- By lowering insulin levels, the Atkins diet stimulates production of C-reactive protein (CRP) in the body, which is a potent inhibitor of inflammation. The risk of inflammation is remarkably decreased. The Atkins diet is an excellent approach to deal with inflammatory conditions like arthritis.

- The Atkins diet is known to reduce the incidence of hypercholesterolemia, gastroesophageal reflux disease (GERD), acne, polycystic ovary syndrome (PCOS), narcolepsy, dementia and certain kinds of cancer. The preventive role of the Atkins diet in these diseases has been proved through extensive research studies.

- Atkins diet favors rapid weight loss. It especially targets abdominal fat stores and reduces their amount, resulting in a better body shape.

- By inducing early satiety and reducing the appetite, people involuntarily end up eating less. This helps with weight loss.

Cons

- 'Ketosis" is one of the inevitable side effects of the Atkins diet, the reason being that the body uses fats for energy production and "ketones" are the products of fat metabolism that are used as energy. Ketosis is an accumulation of excess ketones in the body. This condition is characterized by a particular bad breath, irritability, mood swings, nausea and fatigue. Ketosis only happens when carbohydrates are extremely restricted and too much fat is being burnt down. Since the amount of carbohydrates is increased gradually in the later stages of the plan, ketosis is less likely to develop. If signs and symptoms of ketosis become apparent, slightly lessen the intake of fats while still sticking to the low carb and high protein plan until these symptoms are reversed.

- Sticking to the Atkins diet can mean a complete change in your lifestyle. You'll suddenly find yourself shopping for food in a completely different way. Similarly, people feel quite restricted when it comes to a new diet. The monotony can be quite taxing and your will power to stick to the new dietary regime may start dwindling. Think out of the box and color your menu with the dietary choices that you have. Learn to make new recipes out of the few ingredients (which are not too few, if you go through the full list of foods that the diet allows). By varying the menu every single day, your meals can become something that you look forward to and you can learn to relish them instead of eating merely out of duty. Bring all sorts of vegetables to your meal table and vary the colors. It will also ensure that you are getting your share of all the other essential nutrients like antioxidants and minerals.

Beware!

As I mentioned above, some people tend to suffer from initial side effects when they start a low carb diet. They are, however, completely reversible once the person becomes accustomed to this diet. They include:

- Irritability
- Headaches
- Bad breath due to ketone production
- Weakness
- Palpitations
- Dizziness
- Constipation

This regime is not for you if you are suffering from:

- Kidney disease
- High cholesterol levels
- High blood pressure
- Diabetes
- Heart problems

To help you make sense of what you can eat during beginner phases, I have included the lists of major food groups with net carb count. Pay attention to serving sizes.

Net Crab Lists of Major Food Groups

Aim for 12-15 grams of net carbs per day from vegetables (equal to several cups depending on the carb content). 1 cup is roughly the size of baseball.

Vegetable List

Serving size: ¼ cup, unless otherwise indicated

Vegetable	Net carbs - grams
Alfalfa sprouts (raw, ½ cup)	0.0
Artichoke	6.9
Artichoke marinated (1 each)	1.0
Asparagus	2.4
Beans, green	2.9
Beets	6.5
Bok Choy	0.7

Vegetable	Net carbs - grams
Broccoli	1.7
Brussels Sprouts	7.6
Cabbage	1.1
Carrot	5.1
Cauliflower	1.5
Celery	0.8
Collard Greens	3.0
Corn (1/2 cup)	14.9
Cucumber	1.8
Eggplant	2.0
Endive (raw, ½ cup)	0.1
Escarole (raw, ½ cup)	0.1
Garlic (1 clove)	1.0
Heart of palm (1 each)	0.7
Kale (cooked, ½ cup)	2.4
Lettuce	0.5
Mushroom	1.0
Okra (cooked, ½ cup)	1.8
Olives, green (5 each)	0.1
Olives, black (5 each)	0.7
Onion	4.0
Parsnip	9.0
Peas	6.5

Vegetable	Net carbs - grams
Peppers, green	3.4
Peppers, red	3.3
Pickle (1 medium)	2.0
Portobello mushroom (cooked, 1 each)	2.6
Potato (baked, ½ small)	13.1
Pumpkin	6.3
Radish	0.5
Rutabaga	4.0
Spinach	0.2
Squash, yellow	1.4
Sweet potato (baked, ½ medium)	9.9
Tomato	3.2
Cherry tomato (10 each)	4.6
Turnips	2.3
Zucchini	3.3

Fruit List

Serving size: ¼ cup, unless otherwise indicated

Fruit	Net carbs - grams
Applesauce	6.2
Apple (whole)	17.4
Apricot (whole)	3.1
Avocado (whole)	0.5
Banana (1 small)	20.4
Cantaloupe	3.0
Cherries	4.2
Cherries (1 cup)	17
Clementine (1 each)	7.6
Coconut	1.3
Dates (fresh, 3)	15.8
Dates (chopped)	29.5
Figs, fresh (1 each)	4.5
Grapes	6.7
Grapefruit (1 whole)	9.0
Honeydew	3.6
Kiwi	6.5
Lemon (1 whole)	3.8
Mango	6.3
Orange (1 whole)	12.9

Fruit	Net carbs - grams
Passionfruit (1 whole)	2.0
Papaya ($^1/_2$ cup)	6.6
Peach (1 whole)	8.9
Pear (1 medium)	21
Pineapple	4.3
Plantain	12.0
Plum (1 whole)	7.6
Raisins (1 tbsp)	6.8
Watermelon	2.6

Berry List

Serving size: ¼ cup, unless otherwise indicated

Berry	Net carbs – grams
Acai (1 oz or 28.3 gr)	5.0
Blackberry	2.7
Blackberry 1 cup	10.8
Blueberry	4.1
Blueberry 1 cup	14.6
Cranberry	4.0
Currant	4.0
Elderberry	4.0
Gooseberry	9.0
Raspberry	1.5
Strawberry	1.8

Tips to keep in mind when you don't have the list in front of you: we'll divide vegetables into four groups, depending on what part of the plant they come from.

Leaves (almost zero carbs)

Lettuce, Swiss chard, spinach, herbs etc.

Stems and flowers (very low in carbs)

Asparagus, cauliflower, mushrooms and broccoli.

Fruit (moderate in carbs)

Fruit is the part of the plant that contains seeds: peppers, green beans, tomatoes, all squashes, okra and eggplant. Avocado is a fruit and lower in carbs than others.

Roots (very high in carbs)

Potatoes, sweet potatoes, yams, parsnips and water chestnuts.

However, radish, celery root and carrots are lower in carbs.

Grain List

Grain	Serving Size	Net carbs – grams
Barley (cooked)	½ cup	19.2
Grits (cooked)	½ cup	15.2
Millet (cooked)	½ cup	19.5
Oat bran (raw)	2 tbsp	6.0
Oatmeal (dry, steel cut)	¼ cup	11.5
Oatmeal (dry, rolled)	$^1/_3$ cup	19
Polenta (dry)	2 tbsp	12.5
Rice (brown, cooked)	½ cup	21.2
Wheat bran (raw)	2 tbsp	1.6
Wheat germ	2 tbsp	4.9

Grain	Serving Size	Net carbs – grams
Whole wheat bread	1 slice	10.0
Whole wheat pasta (cooked)	½ cup	16.6

Dairy List

Product	Serving Size	Net carbs – grams
Butter	1 tbsp	0.0
Brie Cheese	1 oz	0.13
Cheddar Cheese	1 oz	0.36
Cottage Cheese	1 cup	6.0
Cream Cheese	1 tbsp	0.39
Eggs	2 large	1.0
Feta Cheese	1 oz	1.16
Goat Cheese	1 oz	0.62
Goat Milk	1 cup	11.0
Gruyer Cheese	1 oz	0.0
Kefir	1 cup	10.4
Mozarella Cheese	1 oz	0.62
Parmesan Cheese	1 oz	0.91
Plain Greek Yogurt	1 cup	9.0

Product	Serving Size	Net carbs – grams
Ricotta Cheese	1 oz	0.86
Sour Cream	1 tbsp	0.61
Swiss Cheese	1 oz	1.51

The Bottom Line

Sticking to one kind of meal plan can be quite difficult. Even more difficult is mustering up the courage to adhere to the new diet. Following low carb and high fat/high protein diet may seem too monumental a task at the beginning, but as you fall into the pattern, you'll notice the difference that it brings into your life. It is relatively easy to follow for vegetarians and even vegans.

Only by taking radical measures to change your diet, can you manage maintaining an ideal body weight and attain that dream fitness goal. The long-term benefits of this dietary approach far outweigh its minor drawbacks and can become the drive that will push you to the very end of your weight loss journey.

GET MOVING:

THE POWER OF WALKING

One of the most common notions about physical exercise is that running or jogging is superior to walking when it comes to losing pounds and staying slim. After all, it's only logical that 45 minutes of running burns off more calories than a 45-minute long walk, BUT you might be wrong here. Recent studies, taken up for the purpose of studying the benefits of walking vs. other exercise regimes like running or jogging, have led scientists to believe that walking has far better outcomes than strenuous running. Walking seems to be the simplest of exercises, yet it has amazing health benefits. This chapter outlines the advantages that accompany walking and busts some popular myths about walking.

How Does Walking Affect Our Body?
A myriad of health benefits are derived from walking.

- **Muscles and joints**

One of the primary benefits of walking is stronger muscles. When muscles remain inactive for a long time, they start wasting away – a process that is scientifically known as "disuse atrophy" of muscles. Their functional capacity reduces. Walking is a great way to kick them back into action so that both muscle bulk and muscle function are improved. Walking mainly affects the leg muscles. In addition, exercise also helps improve functions of joints, ligaments, and tendons. That is why people who walk regularly, even for half an hour every day, are less likely to suffer from joint ailments, especially arthritis.

- **Bones**

It goes without saying that walking is a great way of exercising the bones and improving their density. Walking applies gentle stress on the bones of feet and legs, thereby keeping them structurally and functionally healthy. This is because walking causes bone forming cells to become active and lay down more bone mass, thus strengthening the bones.

- **Weight loss**

Walking at a medium pace can help cut down fat stores of the body, thereby reducing your weight. In overweight people who have trouble running, jogging, or undertaking any other form of physical activity, walking is an easy exercise that can help them decrease their body weight.

- **Cardiovascular benefits**

By reducing cholesterol concentration in the body, walking helps prevent deposition of cholesterol plaque in blood vessels. The vessels are, therefore, less likely to clog and the blood supply to organs, especially the heart and the brain, is prevented from getting compromised. This is how walking helps improve the cardiac profile and lowers the risk of stroke and cardiovascular diseases, especially angina and heart attack. It also helps prevent such diseases as high blood pressure and diabetes.

- **Skin**

As your limbs start moving, blood is directed from the central organs towards the periphery. As the surface blood vessels dilate and blood flows through them more freely, the skin cells get better nutrition, which brings a glow to the skin. This keeps skin fresh and delays the signs of aging – all thanks to walking!

- **Mental health**

By keeping you preoccupied, walking helps banish negative thoughts from your mind. It helps you stay positive by bringing you a sense of doing something worthwhile to change your life. Thereby, walking helps alleviate anxiety and prevents mental ailments like depression.

How Is Walking Better Than Running?

Now we come to the part that you were curious to know about right from the beginning. The foremost reason is psychological impact associated with walking. Walking seems to be much easier to start as compared to any other exercise regime. That is why people are more willing to take up walking. It doesn't even require going to a park, gym or any other specific place. You can even do it in your own backyard or going around the block. A long-term walking routine is, therefore, easier to maintain as compared to a long-term running routine. Even if you plan to undertake a strenuous exercise routine later on, walking helps build up the momentum.

The health benefits of walking have also been proven to be better than running. In order to prove it, researchers at the Life Science Division at Lawrence Berkeley National Laboratory compared the effects of walking to running in about 1,600 subjects. It turned out that the percentage of benefits of walking was higher in terms of preventing hypertension, diabetes, cardiovascular disorders, and reducing cholesterol.

Running also imposes greater stress on joints, especially knees. This causes greater harm than benefit as the joint structures start wearing down. This wear and tear phenomenon can cause early onset of arthritis, especially osteoarthritis. Walking, on the other hand, inflicts less stress and helps improve the joint function instead of deteriorating it.

Running, especially long-distance running has also been proven to place extra stress on the immune system of the body compared to walking. That is why runners are more prone to infections than are walkers. Moreover, as runners are more prone to injuries like sprains, walking is a safer alternative to running.

How To Do it Best?

To make the most of walking every day, it is better to do it the right way. Physical trainers advise people who walk to land on their heels first. The motion should progress from "heel to toe". This helps the push off from the ground to be more powerful while landing on the ball of the foot helps stabilize the body. The net effect is a faster gait.

Walking with an upright posture with the ribcage held slightly in is another recommended technique. Walking with a stoop, it seems, has no effect on the body whatsoever. Pulling the tummy in while walking puts an additional strain on the abdominal muscles and helps strengthen them.

Experts advise to walk at least 10,000 steps on a daily basis. The pace should be medium. It should not be slow enough to be categorized as a stroll; neither should it be as fast as a run. For the purpose of walking, always wear comfortable shoes so that the shock-absorbing function of joints is improved and they do not have to bear additional stress. Wearing uncomfortable shoes is also likely to tire you out quicker. The ideal way, as advised by fitness experts, is to walk for an hour at a medium pace every day to maintain health and a great body shape.

If time is a big limitation for a daily walking routine, you can start with trying alternative techniques like walking a block instead of riding the bus. Climbing a flight of stairs instead of taking the elevator has the same effect. Another great way is to do chores yourself. It'll help you stay healthy. Even if half an hour of walking sounds too much, you can aim for 15 minutes twice a day to start.

Walking is an easy way to stay fit. If you have even 15 minutes on hand, don't spend it lounging around or in front of your TV. Choose to take a walk around the block instead. It'll make you get out of the house and breathe some fresh air too. It's not just a step, it's a step towards a better, healthier future.

EASY RECIPES FOR LIFE:

BREAKFAST, LUNCH AND DINNER

This recipe section is just a road map for you to get started on your weight-loss journey. The majority of the recipes have been adapted from the Atkins program and Nutribullet NutriLiving. They have all been tested and perfected. As a side note, if you're looking for a new blender and are preparing smoothies just for yourself, Nutribullet is a really great option. You don't have to buy Vitamix or Blendtec (however, these are the Ferraris of blenders), any regular blender will do to get you started.

I included only those recipes that are tasty, healthy, nutritious and, at the same time, easy to prepare. These are my daily go-to recipes. Most of the ingredients are the ones you either already have or are easy to find in any grocery store. No cooking experience is required either – preparing your own food should be easy and fun, anyone can do it!

One of my favorite tricks for a snack or a quick breakfast is plain yogurt (Greek yogurt is my favorite for its consistency) with added fruits or berries (fresh or frozen). If you're using frozen treats and leave them to thaw at room temperature, you'll get a sweet syrup along with tasty fruits.

Your yogurt, topped with them, will be so delicious and will have no added sugar! For me, this treat also curbs my ice-cream cravings. For those who absolutely have to have a frozen dessert, I included a simple, one-ingredient (yes, you read this right – one-ingredient) recipe for a banana ice cream. I hope you'll also enjoy a two-ingredient pancake recipe ☺

Enjoy and bon appétit!

BREAKFAST

CHEDDAR OMELET WITH SWISS CHARD AND ONIONS

Ingredients

- 1 tablespoon light olive oil

- 2 cups Swiss chard

- ¼ cup shredded cheddar cheese

- 2 eggs (whole)

- ¼ cup chopped onions

Nutrient count

- Protein - 20.8 grams

- Fat - 32.5 grams

- Fiber - 1.8 grams

Directions

- Pour 2 teaspoons of olive oil in a non-stick pan and heat it on medium heat.

- Add white onions and sauté them till they become tender.

- Immediately add the chard and sauté again till it

wilts.

- Squeeze out water from the chard by pressing it with the spatula. Take it out of the pan, drain and set it aside.

- In the pan, add the remaining olive oil and heat it lightly.

- Add eggs to the pan and let them cook till they become firm on one side. Flip them over and cook the other side.

- Cover half of the omelet with onions and chard and top them with cheese. Cover it with the other half of the omelet.

- Cook for another 2 minutes to melt the cheese.

- Add black pepper and salt to season.

- Serve while still hot.

BAKED TOFU

Ingredients

- 6 oz firm silken tofu

- 1 tsp extra virgin olive oil

Nutrient count

- Protein - 15.1 grams

- Fat - 13.3 grams

- Fiber - 0.5 grams

Directions

- Drain and pat tofu dry with a paper towel. Cut into $1/4$-inch strips. Pour olive oil over tofu. Season with salt and pepper or other seasonings of choice.

- Preheat oven to 375°.

- Bake on a greased flat pan for 15 minutes, turn over and bake an additional 15 minutes till it turns golden brown and slightly crispy.

COCONUT-VANILLA SHAKE

Ingredients

- 1 14 oz can coconut cream

- 2 scoops vanilla whey protein

- ½ tsp vanilla extract

Nutrient count

- Protein - 21.8 grams

- Fat - 23.9 grams

- Fiber - 0.6 grams

Directions

- Place coconut milk, protein powder, vanilla and 2 cups of ice cubes in a blender and pulse until smooth and creamy.

GREEN BREAKFAST POWER SMOOTHIE

<u>Ingredients</u>

- ½ cup spinach

- ½ cup kale

- 1 kiwi

- ¼ cup Greek yogurt

- 1 banana

- 10 grapes

- 1 chunk cucumber

- ½ stalk celery

- ½ apple

- water (1-2 cups, adjusted to the blender)

<u>Directions</u>

- Place all ingredients into your blender and blend for 30 seconds, or until smooth.

BEET BERRY BOUNTY

Ingredients

- 2 cups spinach

- ½ cup blueberries

- 1 cup strawberries

- 1 tablespoon Chia seeds

- ¼ cup almonds

- ¼ cup beets

- 1 cup coconut water

- ½ cup water

Nutrient count

- Protein - 14 grams

- Fat - 22 grams

- Carbs - 43 grams

Directions

- Place all ingredients into your blender and blend for 30 seconds, or until smooth.

BANANA KALE BONANZA

<u>Ingredients</u>

- ½ tall cup kale

- ½ cup mixed berries

- 1 banana

- 1tablespoon hemp seeds

- water

<u>Nutrient count</u>

- Protein - 2.6 grams

- Fat - 7.1 grams

- Carbs - 38.5 grams

- Fiber - 9.2 grams

<u>Directions</u>

- Place all ingredients into your blender and blend for 40 seconds, or until smooth.

ANTI-INFLAMMATORY SUPER CHARGE

<u>Ingredients</u>

- 1 stalk celery

- 1 cup cucumber

- ½ cup pineapple

- ½ lime

- 1 ½ cups coconut water

<u>Nutrient count</u>

- Protein - 4.2 grams

- Fat - 1.7 grams

- Carbs - 31.6 grams

- Fiber - 7.6 grams

<u>Directions</u>

- Place all ingredients into your blender and blend for 40 seconds, or until smooth.

BELL PEPPER RINGS FILLED WITH EGGS AND MOZZARELLA

Ingredients

- ½ medium sweet red pepper

- 2 large eggs (Whole)

- 1 tsp vegetable oil

- ¼ cup shredded mozzarella cheese (whole milk)

Nutrient count

- Protein - 18.7 grams

- Fat - 19.9 grams

- Fiber - 1 grams

Directions

- Cut bell pepper in half across the middle, and then cut two 1-inch rings. Remove seeds and ribs.

- Place rings in sauté pan with oil over medium-high heat. Place an egg in each ring and cook until desired doneness (do not flip).

- Top eggs with cheese, cover and cook 1 more minute until cheese has melted. Season to taste with salt and freshly ground black pepper.

- Serve immediately.

FLUFFY FLAX WAFFLES

Ingredients

- 1/8 cup unsweetened coconut milk

- 2 eggs (whole)

- 1 tablespoon vegetable oil

- 1 teaspoon vanilla extract

- ½ cup organic 100% whole ground golden flaxseed meal

- 1 ounce (vanilla) whey protein - optional

- ½ teaspoon baking powder

- 1 tablespoon sugar free sweetener (ex. Steevia)

- $^1/_8$ teaspoon nutmeg (ground)

- $^1/_8$ teaspoon salt

Nutrient count

- Protein - 22.2 grams

- Fat - 22.5 grams

- Fiber - 2.5 grams

Directions

- Preheat a non-stick waffle maker after spraying it with non-stick spray.

- Combine 2 tablespoons of coconut milk, eggs, oil and vanilla in a small bowl. Blend thoroughly for about 1 minute.

- Add the flax meal, protein powder, baking powder, sweetener, nutmeg and salt. Mix thoroughly for 1-2 minutes.

- Pour half of the batter into the waffle maker.

- Cook for 3-5 minutes until golden brown and set.

- Serve with butter and pancake syrup as desired.

BEEF, SAUTEED WITH GREEN BELL PEPPER AND ONIONS, TOPPED WITH CHEESE

<u>Ingredients</u>

- ¼ cup chopped onions

- 1 tbsp extra virgin olive oil

- ½ cup chopped green sweet pepper

- ½ cup shredded cheddar cheese

- 5 oz ground beef (80% lean / 20% fat)

<u>Nutrient count</u>

- Protein - 43.5 grams

- Fat - 47.1 grams

- Fiber - 2 grams

<u>Directions</u>

- Sauté ground beef in a skillet over medium-high heat with a little bit of cooking oil for 1-2 minutes. Add green bell pepper and white onions.

- Sauté until beef is browned and both peppers and onions are soft. Add salt and pepper to taste.

- Drain off any excess fat and put onto a serving plate. Sprinkle cheese on top and allow to melt. Serve immediately.

EGGS AND SPINACH

Ingredients

- 1 tablespoon extra virgin olive oil

- 2 ½ cup spinach

- 2 eggs (whole)

Nutrient count

- Protein - 13.7 grams

- Fat - 13.9 grams

- Fiber - 1.3 grams

Directions

- Add oil to a non-stick pan and heat it over medium heat.

- Add spinach and sauté until it wilts.

- Add eggs to the pan and scramble together until eggs are cooked.

- Season to taste with salt and freshly ground black pepper before serving.

LUNCH

CRUSTLESS BROCCOLI QUICHE

Ingredients

- 1 teaspoon extra virgin olive oil

- 1 lb broccoli flower clusters

- ½ small onion

- 1 cup cream

- 1 cup shredded cheddar cheese

- 4 eggs (whole)

- ¼ teaspoon thyme

- ¼ teaspoon dried rosemary

- ¼ teaspoon oregano

- ½ teaspoon salt

- ¼ teaspoon black pepper

- ½ cup water

Nutrient count

- Protein - 12 grams

- Fats - 18 grams

- Fiber - 2.1 grams

<u>Directions</u>

- Preheat oven to 375°F.

- Brush a 9" or 10" pie plate with extra virgin olive oil.

- Heat 1 teaspoon of oil in a pan over medium heat.

- Add white onion to the pan and cook for about 2-3 minutes till it becomes soft.

- Transfer into a medium sized bowl and let it cool.

- Add eggs to the onions and beat them lightly.

- Add in ½ cup of cheese, water, thyme, oregano, salt, pepper and rosemary and mix thoroughly.

- Cover the bottom of pie plate with broccoli. Pour egg mixture over it and sprinkle the remaining ½ cup of cheese.

- Bake for about 50 to 60 minutes till a knife inserted in middle comes out clean and quiche is golden brown. The quiche is ready to be served.

ITALIAN FRITTATA

Ingredients

- ½ cup chopped onions

- 1 tablespoon light olive oil

- 1 tablespoon unsalted butter stick

- 1 teaspoon garlic

- 1 large zucchini

- 1 teaspoon dried basil leaves

- 8 oz Italian sausages (raw)

- 2 tablespoon water

- 8 eggs (whole)

- ¼ teaspoon salt

- ¼ teaspoon black pepper

- $1/3$ cup Parmesan cheese (grated)

Nutrient count

- Protein - 24.3g

- Fat - 29.5g

- Fiber -1.2g

Directions

- Preheat broiler.

- Heat the oil and butter in a large, ovenproof skillet over medium heat.

- Add garlic and white onion and sauté for 2 to 3 minutes until softened.

- Add zucchini and basil and cook for 5-6 minutes until soft.

- Add sausage and cook for 2 to 3 minutes, stirring occasionally.

- Meanwhile, in a large bowl whisk together eggs, water, salt and pepper.

- Pour the egg mixture into the hot pan over meat and vegetable mixture.

- Let it cook for a few seconds, undisturbed, then use a spatula to move eggs toward the center while tilting the pan to let the uncooked eggs run to the sides.

- Continue cooking and moving the egg mixture for 4- 5 minutes until eggs are almost set.

- Sprinkle with cheese and place under the broiler until eggs are cooked on top and cheese is melted and bubbly (for about 2-3 minutes).

- Cut in quarters and serve immediately.

AUBERGINE AND RICOTTA ROLLS

Ingredients

- 2 teaspoons black pepper

- 1 teaspoon salt

- 1 teaspoon fresh oregano

- 500 grams whole milk Ricotta cheese

- 4 tablespoons olive oil

- 2 aubergine

Nutrient count

- Protein - 28.6 grams

- Fat - 60.2 grams

- Fiber - 10.3 grams

Directions

- Preheat grill at high temperature.

- Place aubergine on baking tray and brush with oil.

- Cook under preheated grill, about 6cm from the heat source, for 5-6 minutes or until brown.

- Turn and brush with remaining oil.

- Grill for further 2-3 minutes or until tender.

- Meanwhile, combine ricotta and oregano in a medium bowl.

- Season with salt and pepper.

- Spoon ricotta mixture evenly among aubergine slices and roll to enclose.

- Place the rolls on serving plates and sprinkle with oregano leaves to garnish.

CAULIFLOWER CRUST PIZZA

Adopted from the LuckyPennyBlog web-site

Makes a 10-12 inch pizza

<u>Ingredients</u>

- 1 small to medium sized head of cauliflower (should yield 2 to 3 cups once processed)

- ¼ teaspoon kosher salt

- ½ teaspoon dried basil (crush it even more between your fingers)

- ½ teaspoon dried oregano (crust it even more between your fingers)

- ½ teaspoon garlic powder

- ¼ cup shredded parmesan cheese

- ¼ cup mozzarella cheese

- 1 egg

Optional:

- 1 tablespoon almond meal

- a few shakes of crushed red pepper

<u>Directions</u>

- Preheat oven to 450 degrees. On a cutting board, place a large piece of parchment paper and spray it with nonstick cooking oil. Place a baking sheet or a pizza stone in the oven.

- Wash and thoroughly dry a small head of cauliflower.

- Cut off the florets. Pulse in a food processor for about 30 seconds, until you get powdery "snow-like" cauliflower. You should end up with 2 to 3 cups cauliflower "snow". Instead of food processor you can use cheese grater to grate the cauliflower.

- Place cauliflower in a microwave safe bowl and cover. Microwave for 4 minutes. Instead of microwaving, you can steam it just enough to get it slightly tender. Place cooked cauliflower onto a clean towel and allow to cool before the next step.

- Once cauliflower is cool enough to handle, wrap it up in the dish towel and wring it. You want to squeeze out as much water as possible. This will ensure you get a chewy pizza-like crust.

- Place cauliflower in a bowl. It will almost look like flour! Now add $^1/_4$ cup parmesan cheese, $^1/_4$ cup mozzarella cheese, $^1/_4$ teaspoon kosher salt, $^1/_2$ teaspoon dried basil, $^1/_2$ teaspoon dried oregano, $^1/_2$ teaspoon garlic powder and a dash of red pepper if you want. Add almond meal if you have closer to 2 cups of cauliflower "snow" (don't add if you have closer to 3 cups as that'll be enough). Now add an egg and mix.

- Once mixed together, use your hands to form the dough into a crust on your oiled parchment paper. Pat it down thoroughly, you want it tightly formed together. Don't make it too thick or too thin.

- Using a cutting board, slide the parchment paper onto your hot pizza stone or baking sheet in the oven. Bake for 8 - 11 minutes.

- Take the pizza out to add sauce and toppings. However, go off looks rather than time as different ovens may cook differently! You want the edges to be crispy brown but not too much, so that when you cook it again after adding toppings it won't burn.

- Now add the sauce, cheese and toppings you want.

- Slide parchment with topped pizza back into the hot oven and cook for another 5 to 7 minutes until the cheese is melted, bubbly and slightly golden.

- Allow to cool for two minutes. Then, using a pizza cutter and a spatula serve up your delicious grain-free cauliflower crust pizza!

HOMEMADE PIZZA SAUCE

Adopted from the LuckyPennyBlog web-site

Makes about 16oz

<u>Ingredients</u>

- 1 ½ teaspoon olive oil

- ½ small to medium onion, diced

- 3 - 4 garlic cloves, minced

- 2 8oz cans no salt tomato sauce

- ½ teaspoon sugar

- 1 teaspoon dried oregano

- 1 teaspoon dried basil

- ½ to 1 teaspoon kosher salt

- ½ teaspoon garlic powder

<u>Directions</u>

- Heat 1 $^1/_2$ teaspoons olive oil in a pot over medium heat. Once hot, add the diced onion. Sauté until soft, about 4 minutes.

- Add garlic and sauté for another 2 minutes. Garlic should be golden and fragrant and onions should be soft.

- Add tomato sauce to the pot and all seasonings; stir.

- Once sauce begins to bubble, reduce heat to medium low. Let cook for at least 15 minutes, longer if you have time or while you prep and cook your pizza crust.

- Store in an airtight container with a lid.

DINNER

HERBED SMOKED SALMON IN TOMATO HALVES

Ingredients

- 2 medium sized tomatoes

- ½ teaspoon extra-virgin olive oil

- ½ teaspoon Herbs de Provence

- 5 beaten eggs

- 4oz smoked salmon, roughly chopped

- 1 tablespoon cream-cheese

- 2 tablespoons chopped fresh chives

- 1 teaspoon grated Parmesan cheese

Nutrient count

- Protein - 13.6g

- Fat - 8.8g

- Fiber - 0.5g

Directions

- Preheat broiler.

- Cut tomatoes in half and scoop out seeds.

- Drizzle each half with a little bit of olive oil and sprinkle with herbs.

- Broil for about 3 minutes to heat tomatoes. Turn off broiler and close the oven door.

- Meanwhile, in a medium skillet over medium heat, scramble the eggs. Before they are set, add salmon, cream cheese and chives.

- Remove tomatoes from oven and fill each with one-quarter of the egg mixture.

- Sprinkle with cheese and serve.

ASIAN TUNA SALAD

Ingredients

- 175gr tuna fillet

- 3 pieces bok choy

- 30gr tinned water chestnuts

- 6 radishes

- 1 tomato

- 1 tablespoon soya sauce

Nutrient count

- Protein -72.4g

- Fat - 14.2g

- Fiber - 6.1 g

Directions

- Grill the tuna and steam the bok choy.

- Stir fry with the rest of the ingredients in soya sauce.

CARBONARA PENNE

Ingredients

- 2 packs bacon

- 30 ml cream

- 1 egg (whole)

- ½ clove garlic

- 1 teaspoon salt

- 1 teaspoon black pepper

- 1 teaspoon fresh parsley

- 25 gr penne pasta

Nutrient count

- Proteins - 27.1 g

- Fat - 16.1 g

- Fiber - 7.4 g

Directions

- Boil water in a saucepan and add 25g penne per person and cook until soft.

- Meanwhile, cut the bacon into strips and fry until lightly golden.

- Add crushed garlic and parsley and cook for a few seconds, then remove from heat and set aside.

- Drain the pasta and add to the frying pan with other ingredients.

- Add the beaten egg and half of the grated cheese.

- Season with salt & pepper and mix.

- Put into a serving dish and sprinkle with the rest of the cheese.

SNACKS AND DESSERTS

CHOCOLATE HAZELNUT SMOOTHIE

Ingredients

- 2 scoops chocolate whey protein

- 1 tablespoon heavy cream

- 12 tablespoons sugar-free hazelnut syrup

Nutrient count

- Protein - 23.2 grams

- Fat - 22.2 grams

- Fiber - 0 gram

Directions

- Add whey protein, cream and hazelnut syrup to a blender.

- Add ice.

- Blend till it becomes smooth.

- Pour into glasses and top with cinnamon powder.

APPLE MUFFINS WITH CINNAMON-PECAN STREUSEL

<u>Ingredients</u>

- 1 2/3 cups almond meal flour

- ½ cup pecan halves

- 6 ½ teaspoons cinnamon

- 1/3 teaspoon salt

- 24 teaspoons erythritol

- 1 pinch of stevia

- 2 tablespoons unsalted butter stick

- 2 eggs (whole)

- ¼ cup unsweetened coconut milk

- 2 teaspoons vanilla extract

- ½ cup organic high fiber coconut flour

- 1 teaspoon baking powder

- $^2/_3$ cup quartered or chopped apple

<u>Nutrient count</u>

- Protein - 7.5g

- Fat - 20.6g

- Fiber - 5.1g

<u>Directions</u>

- Preheat oven to 350 F.

- Prepare a muffin tin with 8 cupcake papers.

- Combine $^2/_3$ cup almond flour, chopped pecans, 2 tablespoons cinnamon, $^1/_8$ teaspoon salt, 2 tablespoons granular sugar substitute, a pinch of stevia and 2 tablespoons melted butter in a small bowl. Mix with a fork until it begins to crumble. Set aside while making the muffin batter.

- For the muffins: whisk together the eggs, $^1/_4$ cup coconut milk, 2 teaspoons vanilla, 6 tablespoons granular sugar substitute, a pinch of stevia, and $^1/_2$ teaspoon ground cinnamon. Add 1 cup almond flour, 2 tablespoons coconut flour, $^1/_4$ teaspoon salt and 1 teaspoon baking powder; mix to combine then fold in $^2/_3$ cup finely chopped apples.

- Divide into 8 muffin wells, topping each with about 2 tablespoons of the streusel.

- Bake for 25 minutes, remove from oven and allow to sit for 10-20 minutes to cool before removing.

- Serve immediately or refrigerate.

PEANUT BUTTER GRANOLA BAR PARFAIT WITH YOGURT AND STRAWBERRIES

Ingredients

- ½ cup plain yogurt

- 5 large strawberries

Nutrient count

- Protein - 24.1g

- Fat - 9.5g

- Fiber - 6.8g

Directions

- In a parfait glass, layer the granola bar (chopped) with yogurt and strawberries.

- The granola bar is ready to be enjoyed.

ONE-INGREDIENT BANANA ICE CREAM

Ingredients

- 1 large ripe banana (sweet and soft)

  Mix-in ideas:

- 1 spoon of peanut butter

- Drizzle of honey

- Chocolate chips

- Almonds

- 1 tablespoon of cocoa powder

- Half a teaspoon of cinnamon or ginger

Directions

- Peel the bananas and cut them into more or less evenly sized coins (don't worry about shape or size in general).

- Put the banana pieces into an airtight container (a freezer-safe glass bowl or a freezer bag).

- Freeze the banana pieces for at least 2 hours (ideally overnight).

- Blend the frozen banana pieces in a small food processor or powerful blender (pulse the pieces, small food processor works best for this).

- Keep blending until you have creamy, soft serve ice cream texture: at first the pieces will look crumbly, then gooey, after that like oatmeal and then the magic will happen.

- Blend for a few more seconds to aerate the ice cream.

- If you'd like to add some chocolate chips or peanut butter – this is the time to do it.

- Transfer to an airtight container and freeze until solid (you can eat this ice cream immediately, of course, but it will be quiet soft).

TWO-INGREDIENT BANANA PANCAKES

Makes 8 small pancakes, easily doubled

Ingredients

- 1 medium ripe banana

- 2 large eggs

   Optional extras (chose a few):

- $^1/_8$ teaspoon baking powder – for fluffier pancakes
- $^1/_8$ teaspoon salt
- ¼ teaspoon vanilla
- 1 tablespoon cocoa powder
- 1 tablespoon honey
- ½ cup chopped nuts, chocolate chips or a mix
- 1 cup fresh fruit or berries
- Coconut oil or butter for the pan
- Maple syrup or honey for topping

Directions

- Peel the banana, break it up and mash with a fork in a bowl. Continue until it has a pudding-like consistency (a few small lumps are ok).

- Add any extra ingredients – but these pancakes are great on their own.

- Whisk the eggs together until yolks and whites are completely combined. Pour the eggs over the banana and stir until the eggs are completely combined. The batter will be liquid and it's ok.

- Heat a pan with a little bit of butter or coconut oil to prevent sticking, if you'd like.

- Use around 2 tablespoons of batter per pancake – it should sizzle immediately (if not, slightly turn up the heat).

- Cook the pancakes until the bottom is brown and golden – around 1 minute.

- Sprinkle any loose toppings as the first side cooks.

- Gently work the spatula about halfway under the pancake, then lift until the other half is just barely lifted. Lay the pancake back down on its opposite side. If any loose batter spills, be sure to put the pancake on top of the spill.

- Cook for another minute or so, until the other side is also golden-brown.

- Transfer the cooked pancakes to the serving plate and continue cooking the rest of the batter. If you're cooking more than a single batch, keep the pancakes warm in the oven.

- Pancakes are best when eaten fresh and warm. Serve with nay extra toppings you'd like.

- Leftovers can be kept in the fridge for a few days and make a great snack.

EAT THIS, NOT THAT:

HEALTHY SUBSTITUES FOR YOUR MUST-HAVE JUNK FOODS

In a perfect world, we would eat whatever we want and stay healthy and fit. But we don't live in a perfect world and eating junk foods comes with its repercussions. The deep fried, chemically induced, overly sweet and high carb fast foods may taste great but they are definitely not healthy. Despite the recent surge in health awareness and body transformation trends, we still have an alarming obesity rate. Junk foods definitely play a big part in that.

Junk foods are the ultimate enemy. They taste great, are extremely convenient, and are also cheaper than good healthy products. However, they are a big threat to your health. When tempted by junk food, remember – your stomach isn't a waste basket!

I understand that it is not easy to stop eating junk food at once. So to make the transition easier for you, I bring you some of the most popular junk foods and their healthy alternatives. Also, keep in mind that if you keep good food in your fridge and around the house, you will eat good food.

Burger
Without a doubt, burgers are the number one junk food. They are loved by people of all ages. Thanks to a burger franchise, opening almost every few miles, these are the most difficult to avoid. A healthier alternative will be to use a whole grain bun, lots of salad and veggies with steam-cooked lean meat. This will be low in calories and high in vitamins, proteins and other vital nutrients. Veggie burgers made with black beans are a perfectly delicious alternative as well.

French Fries
You can ask a bunch of people and not one of them will tell you that they don't like fries. Fries are one of the most popular junk foods across the globe. Instead of frying them in regular cooking oil, try to bake them in coconut oil. This will allow you to get all the nutritious goodness of coconut oil and your fries will still be crunchy and crispy with a beautiful texture. An air fryer is a great alternative to using oil.

Pizza
Another top contender on the list of most popular junk food is pizza. Since originating from the traditional kitchens of Italy, pizza has evolved into several specialties, depending on different regions and recipes. You can alternate the topping of your pizza with healthy vegetables, like eggplants, zucchini, mushrooms, etc. Also, try using a cauliflower crust to avoid excessive carb intake (see delicious recipe in a previous chapter).

Mac & Cheese
Mac & Cheese is a typical all-American junk food, liked and enjoyed by millions across the nation. It's easy to make and delicious, which makes it a widely popular junk food. Instead of using the orange stuff that comes in the box from the supermarket and elbow macaroni, try using butternut

squash. This will add a great texture to your dish and give it a sweet touch.

Ice Cream

The almighty of all the sweet junk foods is the ice cream. This amazing sweet flavored treat is a big health hazard. It contains enormous amounts of sugar, preservatives, artificial sweeteners, and colorants. A great alternative to your regular ice cream is a yogurt and berries treat (where you add the berries and fruits) or a scrumptious one-ingredient banana ice cream. Vegan ice creams are also easy to find in stores and they are low in calories, as they are made from blended frozen fruits. Try one today!

Soda

In my opinion, this is the worst offender of them all. While providing no nutritional benefits at all, it's packed with sugar and chemical additives. It doesn't even quench your thirst! On the contrary, it makes you drink more and more of the same soda and fuels your appetite for other junk food. The invention of soda was a real jackpot by fast food companies. Next time you are tempted to have just one can of soda, think about this little fun fact: the added sugar in a single can of soda might be more than most people would have consumed in an entire year just a few hundred years ago! Stick to pure water instead. Try adding berries or lemon juice to add flavor.

FREQUENTLY ASKED QUESTIONS

1. How long does each phase last?

There's no firm rule to follow but these are the general recommendations to keep in mind:

- **Phase I** – at least 2 weeks; more if you have a lot of excess weight or want to lose extra pounds rather quickly.

- **Phase II** – also at least 2 weeks, but here your weight should be your guide. Transition to Phase III when you're within 10lbs of your desired goal.

- **Phase III** – until you've reached your weight goal plus 1 month of maintenance.

- **Phase IV** – lifetime maintenance – this is the beginning of your new life-style. Congratulations, you did it!

2. I've been on various diets before, they don't last and I always gain my weight back and even more. How exactly is this plan different?

This is not a fad diet that lasts a few weeks that leaves you completely malnourished and starving. This is a well-balanced plan, designed to keep you satiated and nourished, so that your body gets all the proper nutrition you need. Of course, there will be some discomfort and hunger initially, but eventually you'll get used to eating less and feeling stronger and healthier. This is the plan that will teach you how to eat right for life, not just for the duration of your "diet".

3. I work out 5-7 days a week and I seem to bulk up more instead of slimming down. What am I doing wrong?

This is a good one. You would think the more you work out, the more fat you'll burn. This is not always the case. There is such thing as overtraining. If you work out a lot without sufficient rest, this will increase your appetite. Your body will need extra fuel to be able to perform. Furthermore, very often people give themselves permission (subconsciously) to eat more after an intensive workout as they believe they just burned off a lot of calories and sped up their metabolism. For the most part, we also think we burned off many more calories than we really did. In this case, I'd advise to switch to working out 3-4 days a week and staying physically active during the other days. If you run every day and feel this is hindering your weight loss, start walking instead. Walking is a great way to lose weight, especially to slim down and lose weight, provided you spend at least 1 hour a day walking. Be careful here, I'm not talking about a stroll through the park or window shopping ☺ You should walk in a medium to fast pace. Walking won't leave you famished, it will provide a great time for you to relax and gather your thoughts; it can even boost creativity.

4. I hate working out or I'm not in good shape to exercise. Will I still lose weight?

Yes, you will! Being active is so much more than working out and dripping sweat. The key is to be active every day: park your car further away, take stairs instead of the elevator, go for a walk on your lunch break and in the morning (and/or evening). Before we run, we should focus on walking. There's a lot of literature on how walking can help shed extra pounds and get you in the best shape of your life. In this book, I provided general direction to get you started (please also see the question above).

5. I was following the program for a week (two, three, etc.) and then I fell off the wagon – I went back to my old eating habits for a few days (a week, etc.). Is everything lost?

We're all human and this happens even to the best and the strongest of us. It's not the end of the world. Recognize that you slipped mainly because of your old habits – after all, how long have you been eating this way? Change doesn't happen overnight and the occasional slip up will not negate your progress. Even if you gave in and ate a doughnut for breakfast, don't give yourself permission to keep eating bad foods because the day has already been ruined. No, you can get back on track at any moment and it will only make you stronger. The longer you stick with the plan, the easier it will get. And it's ok if it takes you longer than other people.

6. **I love French fries, ice cream, etc. (insert your favorite junk food) and can't imagine living without them.**

Life is about enjoyment and enjoying your food. It's unrealistic to expect anyone to eat bland foods in the name of health and healthy weight. This is why I included some genius tips and recipes how to give your favorite junk food a makeover and still enjoy it without sacrificing your health. Refer to the Chapter "Eat This, Not That".

7. **I need to lose only 5-10lbs. Should I still start the program from Phase 1?**

In this case, you should first analyze your eating habits and your diet. If you eat lots of junk food, drink soda or have mostly a carbohydrate rich diet, for example, tips from the chapters "Stop Counting Calories and Eat More" and "Eat This, Not That" will be sufficient to start. Apply those suggestions and I'm sure those few extra pounds will melt with no other effort. However, if your weight is stuck at the same number, track your physical activity level: do you spend hours sitting behind the desk, driving everywhere and slouching on the couch after a long day at work? It's true that losing 5-10lbs is more difficult than losing more extra weight initially, but following these principles will help you reach your goal.

8. **I've heard so much about losing only water weight in the beginning. Should I limit amount of liquids in my daily diet to speed up my weight loss?**

While you may count tea (especially herbal tea) and broth towards the recommended 8 glasses of water per day, depending on how active you are you might even need more. Don't skimp on hydration in attempt to see a lower number on your scale!

9. **Should I weigh myself daily or weekly to track my progress?**

Don't become a slave to the scale! Since your weight varies slightly from day to day, weighing weekly is the best strategy. Even better – just measure yourself and track your progress. Sometimes that is a better indicator of our progress since transformed muscles may weigh the same but overall you will look much slimmer and fit into clothes of smaller size. Remember, 1lb of fat does not equal1lb of muscle!

10. **Any additional tips you could give me?**

Use a journal to track your progress. I can't stress enough how important this is. Having a daily visual reminder keeps you accountable and motivated. Writing down what you eat daily also helps to see if you're consuming too many carbs or calories in general. On the days when you feel like there hasn't been any progress at all, you will see that there actually was.

BIBLIOGRAPHY

1. Am J Clin Nutr. 2010 Mar; 91(3):535-46. doi: 10.3945/ajcn.2009.27725. Epub 2010 Jan 13. Meta-analysis of prospective cohort studies evaluating the association of saturated fat with cardiovascular disease. Siri-Tarino PW1, Sun Q, Hu FB, Krauss RM.

2. Cochrane Database Syst Rev. 2015 Jun 10;6:CD011737. doi: 10.1002/14651858.CD011737. Reduction in saturated fat intake for cardiovascular disease. Hooper L, Martin N, Abdelhamid A, Davey Smith G.

3. Food Nutr Res. 2014 Jul 10;58. doi: 10.3402/fnr.v58.25145. eCollection 2014. Effect of the amount and type of dietary fat on cardiometabolic risk factors and risk of developing type 2 diabetes, cardiovascular diseases, and cancer: a systematic review. Schwab U1, Lauritzen L2, Tholstrup T2, Haldorssoni T3, Riserus U4, Uusitupa M5, Becker W6.

4. J Eval Clin Pract. 2012 Feb; 18(1):159-68. doi: 10.1111/j.1365-2753.2011.01767.x. Epub 2011 Sep 25. Is the use of cholesterol in mortality risk algorithms in clinical guidelines valid? Ten years prospective data from the Norwegian HUNT 2 study. Petursson H, Sigurdsson JA, Bengtsson C, Nilsen TI, Getz L.

5. Lunn J and Theobald H. (2006) The health effects of dietary unsaturated fatty acids. Nutrition Bulletin 31:178-224

6. Simopoulos A. (2008) The importance of the omega-6/omega-3 fatty acid ratio in cardiovascular disease and other chronic diseases. Experimental Biology and

Medicine. Published online 11 April 2008. DOI:10.3181/0711-MR-311

7. Atkins R. C, MD "Atkins for Life"

8. Atkins R. C., MD "Dr. Atkin's Age Defying Diet"

9. Hyman M., MD "The Ultramind Solution"

10. Hyman M., MD "The Blood Suga Solution"

Take a minute to leave a review on Amazon,

letting me know what you have learned from this book.

I always want to hear from my readers and know how your healthy lifestyle is going.

Thank you ☺

NOTES

NOTES

www.ingramcontent.com/pod-product-compliance
Lightning Source LLC
Chambersburg PA
CBHW050035260726

48658CB00005B/1620